HERBAL REMEDIES

RHEUMATISM & ARTHRITIS

MERVYN A. MITTON

W. Foulsham & Company Limited
London · New York · Toronto · Cape Town · Sydney

KV-748-545

W. Foulsham & Company Limited
Yeovil Road, Slough, Berkshire, SL1 4JH

ISBN 0-572-01242-X

Copyright © 1984 Mervyn Mitton

All rights reserved.
The Copyright Act (1956) prohibits (subject to certain very
limited exceptions) the making of copies of any copyright
work or of a substantial part of such a work, including
the making of copies by photocopying or similar process.
Written permission to make a copy or copies must therefore
normally be obtained from the publisher in advance. It is
advisable also to consult the publisher if in any doubt as
to the legality of any copying which is to be undertaken.

Designed and Illustrated by Gecko Studio Services
Phototypeset in Great Britain by Input Typesetting Ltd,
London and printed by St Edmundsbury Press,
Bury St Edmunds, Suffolk

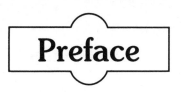

Preface

During the early years of this century, by far the greatest majority of medicinal remedies available were based on herbal materials and, in fact, many of the formulae prescribed by doctors were the ones used with success in past centuries. Even as late as the 1940s, it would probably be true to say that at least fifty per cent of a doctor's prescriptions would still have herbal materials contained in them.

During the sixties and seventies, the medical profession appeared to discard all of the older, proven methods of treatment in favour of new chemical based drugs. The results of this revised thinking can be read about weekly in the newspapers when they report side-effects – many of them very serious – from so many of these new and relatively untested medicines.

Within the last few years, however, there has been a dramatic resurgence of interest, both from the medical profession and the general public, in alternative forms of medicine – particularly herbs – and this book will help you to find your way through the many possibilities for safe home treatment. As a consulting herbalist at Cathay of Bournemouth, a firm established by my parents many years ago and now the largest retail herbalists in Britain, I can offer information and advice which is totally relevant and current.

Contents

Introduction

During the Second World War – and even today in some research laboratories and American prisons – human guinea pigs were used to test new drugs and their effect on the human system. The inducements for taking these risks were usually either a payment, or in the case of prisoners, a remission of their sentence.

Unfortunately, no freedom of choice or inducements have been made to the many thousands of unfortunate patients who, over the last few years, have been subjected to an unintentional 'guinea pig' testing of new arthritic and rheumatic drugs some of which have obviously been launched in advance of a complete knowledge of their safety. I refer specifically to Opren and Osmosin, both of which have recently been suspended by the Committee on the Safety of Medicines.

From medical reports currently available, it would seem that Opren has been held to have been responsible for over 60 deaths and over 3,500 patients reported adverse side-effects including nausea, dyspepsia, vomitting, haemorrhaging, nail separation, headaches and sun-sensitivity.

Similar reports show that Osmosin could have been responsible for as many as fifteen deaths and with over 400 adverse side-effects reported at the time of its suspension. Side-effects seem to have been mainly severe headaches and gastro-intestinal problems, including haemorrhaging.

Another anti-inflammatory drug, Flosint, has also had its licence revoked. Of 10,000 patients taking the drug,

217 are thought to have suffered side-effects such as upset stomach, stomach ulcer irritation and internal bleeding, and for some, dizziness and headaches.

Since rheumatoid arthritis and osteo-arthritis have such serious and debilitating effects, it is not surprising that so many drugs have been tried over the years to alleviate the symptoms. However, many of these drugs have had side-effects and in some cases these have been more serious than the condition they have been attempting to treat! In addition to prescribed drugs listed later, must be considered the potentionally serious side-effect of pain-killers such as Distalgesic, Paracetamol and Aspirin.

Before I am accused of attacking the medical profession indiscriminately, I would like to point out that there are many safe alternative herbal tablets and infusions which can be used for the same anti-inflammatory purposes but with few, if any, of the side-effects. Herbal medicine has never been in opposition to the medical profession, but is rather the original and alternative method of treating illness by natural means, rather than chemical. With the side-effects possible from some of the chemical drugs, I believe it is sensible to look at safer alternatives in the first instance, before taking such potentially serious risks.

That there is a need for help and advice for both men and women troubled by rheumatism and arthritis is obvious – and that this should be based on the known qualities of herbs is equally reasonable, since in many cases they can be easily prepared or taken at home. This home treatment is necessary, since experience has shown that many people wish to try first to control their problem themselves.

This should not mean that where a serious medical condition exists that it should be treated at home from the advice given in this book. In such a case, you should always contact your doctor immediately. However, where the pattern of the problem matches examples given, and where the advice is applicable, then herbal treatment could well be the answer.

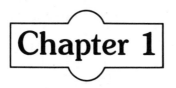

Chapter 1

Identifying your illness

Most people suffering a rheumatic or arthritic condition will have sought medical advice and have had a correct diagnosis made of their particular problem. Sometimes, however, further complications arise, or the condition is not thought serious enough to worry the doctor, and it is for this reason that I show the various forms of these illnesses and their symptoms.

Many of the readers of this book will be dedicated already to the use of natural medicines, others will be seeking alternative treatments to conventional chemical medicines which they may have tried without success. The important thing to remember is that first you must be sure that you have correctly identified the problem – wrong diagnosis could possibly mean a worsening of the condition. Secondly, remember that herbal treatment is relatively slow acting and generally relies on a gradual build-up in the system. This makes it particularly suitable for long-term problems such as arthritis and rheumatism, since herbs are usually without side-effects, not addictive, and compatible with each other.

RHEUMATISM

This is a name applied generally to diseases which have inflammation or degenerative action on the muscles, joints and other parts of the body. The various forms of this illness can usually be summarised as follows.

ACUTE RHEUMATISM
More usually known as rheumatic fever, this is a disease more common in young people and is a recurring one. This condition requires medical treatment.

NON-ARTICULAR RHEUMATISM
Usually of a muscular nature, there are a number of common illnesses which come under this category and are often known as muscular rheumatism. Most have in common a tendency to become worse in cold, damp weather and show improvement when it is warmer.

Many herbs have been found to be of benefit for these conditions. Also the application of gentle heat can bring comfort together with mild exercise and warm clothing.

ASSOCIATED CONDITIONS

Some of the associated conditions of rheumatism are described below.

BURSITIS
These are inflammations within the 'pocket' areas in the body at points where there is a lot of movement. They are most common at elbows, knees and also at the shoulder, giving rise to the painful 'frozen shoulder'. Housemaid's knee and tennis elbow are two common names given when the inflammation is localised. Massage with a good rheumatic balm will often give relief.

FIBROSITIS
This is another name to refer to the condition of muscular rheumatism, particularly when inflammation puts pressure on the endings of the sensory nerves.

LUMBAGO

Lumbago is usually seated in the muscles of the back, particularly when they have been subjected to strain or damage. Sometimes linked with rheumatic attacks in other parts of the body, lumbago often has pain of a sharp stabbing type and can be very incapacitating.

MYALGIA

This is a medical term used to describe muscular pain.

NEURITIS

An inflammation of the nerves, this can be of a restrictive nature as with sciatica attacks.

SCIATICA

A common complaint, sufferers of sciatica usually have it as a result of a slipped back disc pressing on the sciatic nerve. The pain generally runs down through the buttocks into the back of the leg and sometimes into the foot – the side affected depends on where the pressure from the disc is being applied.

GOUT

For years, sufferers of gout have been figures of fun – perhaps because it is usually associated with good living, and therefore in less affluent times was felt to be deserved!

More prone to attack those above middle years, gout's principal nature is an excess of uric acid in the system, which can lay down deposits of urate of soda in the joints. The reason for this excess of acid is not known, but high living in the form of rich food and too much alcohol can be contributory factors. Gout can be hereditary.

Symptoms of an attack of gout can be stomach upsets, liver and sometimes bladder disturbance and eventually very sharp pain – often in the ball of the great toe, but sometimes in the heel or thumb. The affected part swells and takes on a deep red colour. Usually the pain lessens after a few hours, but the normal pattern is for it to return nightly for a week to ten days – the usual period of an attack.

Gout is one of the most painful of the conditions dealt with in this book and being of a degenerative nature, always presents problems.

RHEUMATOID ARTHRITIS

This illness is one which tends to first attack in the years around forty and is more common in women than men. Of all the forms of rheumatism, this is one of the most serious and crippling.

Onset of the disease is generally noticed by pain and swellings in the fingers and this may eventually spread throughout the joints of the body. Rheumatoid arthritis attacks are usually accompanied by a fever, and if the attack is serious the fever can be of equally serious proportions.

The characteristic appearance of the hands is a pulling of the fingers towards the small finger and an enlargement of the joints with wasting of the muscles in between.

Rest, gentle exercise and heat are all of benefit in a general regimen of treatment which should include use of some of the recommended herbs.

OSTEO-ARTHRITIS

Present in a high proportion of older people, this joint disorder is often brought about by pre-existing injury – although it is sometimes thought to be hereditary.Osteo-arthritis is a degenerative condition, but is characterised by periods of remission which can often cause confusion when they occur during times of medical treatment.

The action of the condition is to gradually destroy the central part of the cartilage of the affected joint – and at the same time the outer part grows over the joint. Eventually, bony spurs, known as osteophytes, occur.

Osteo-arthritis most commonly affects the joints of the shoulder, hip and knee and also the end joints of the fingers.

Rest, gentle exercise and heat are of benefit in this condition and, of course, treatment by use of the appropriate herbs. When excess weight is a problem this should be eliminated by dieting to take pressure off the affected joints. Diet can also play an important part in treatment.

Chapter 2

Some commonly used drugs

This chapter outlines some main chemical drugs used in the treatment of rheumatism and arthritis, together with some of their side-effects. This information is not given to frighten people on these drugs, but to make them aware of all of their possible effects – however it should also be realised that not everyone taking a drug will necessarily suffer side-effects.

I believe that many doctors fail to explain fully to their patients the side-effects that can be expected from a particular drug or course of treatment, and this can cause great distress. This is usually a failure of communication since most drug companies advise doctors of the side-effects to be expected from their particular medicines.

Whilst there are other drugs used for rheumatic and arthritic problems which are not on the list, and which are held to have less severe side-effects, it should be remembered that all chemical based drugs are expected to have side-effects.

Proprietary brand names are given in brackets beneath drug name.

BENORYLATE
(Benoral)

May cause gastro-intestinal disturbance and increase the effect of some other drugs.

CORTISONE
(Cortelan)
(Cortisyl)

Side-effects may include hypertension, oedema, mental disturbance, and increased risk of infection.

DIFLUNISAL
(Dolobid)

May cause gastro-intestinal disturbance.

FENCLOFENAC
(Flenac)

May cause gastro-intestinal disturbance.

FENOPROFEN
(Fenopron)

May cause dizziness, nausea, or intestinal disturbance.

FLUFENAMIC ACID
(Arlef)

May cause gastro-intestinal disturbance.

FLURBIPROFEN
(Froben)

Care necessary for stomach ulcer sufferers and some asthmatics.

IBUPROFEN
(Brufen)

Care necessary for stomach ulcer sufferers, some asthmatics and patients with liver problems.

INDOMETHACIN
(Indocid)
(Imbrilon)

May cause headaches, nausea, dyspepsia and some blood disorders.

KETOPROFEN
(Orudis)

Care necessary for patients with ulcer and liver problems. Also some other specialised conditions.

MEFENAMIC ACID
(Ponstan)

May cause gastro-intestinal disturbance.

NAPROXEN
(Naprosyn)

Care necessary for stomach ulcer sufferers.

OXYPHENBUTAZONE
(Tanderil)

Many dangerous side-effects.

PHENYLBUTAZONE
(Butazolidin)

May cause gastro-intestinal disturbance and many other side-effects.

PREDNISONE
(Decortisyl)
(Deltacortone)

May cause gastro-intestinal disturbance and even bring about formation of peptic ulcers.

PREDNISOLONE
(Codelcortone)
(Deltacortril)
(Prednesol)

May cause gastro-intestinal disturbance and even bring about formation of peptic ulcers.

SODIUM AUROTHIOMALATE
(Injections of a gold compound)

Many side-effects, some of them severe.

SODIUM SALICYLATE

Possibility of tinnitus, nausea and other gastro-intestinal disturbances.

SULINDAC
(Clinoril)

May cause gastro-intestinal disturbance and internal bleeding.

TRIAMCINOLONE
(Adcortyl)
(Ledercort)

Some general side-effects are possible.

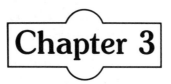

Chapter 3

Some problems which trouble sufferers

One of the worst aspects of rheumatism and arthritis, apart from the pain involved, is their ability to incapacitate by malforming of the hands and limbs. This can lead to people having to give up their jobs and to the discontinuing of favourite hobbies such as sewing and knitting.

There can be no doubt that one of the greatest steps in recent years to help patients has been the technique of plastic joint replacement, and this has given mobility back to many sufferers who had become confined to wheelchairs, or dependent on sticks. However, merely to replace an affected part does not stop the onset of the condition and with the 'growing over' process of arthritis, many people have found changes even of the artificial joints necessary. Therefore, it can be seen that internal control of the factors causing the progression of the illness become all-important.

Whilst causes leading to the start of these illnesses can often be pin-pointed, it is still not generally understood why some people are more prone than others – or why a more marked and rapid deterioration occurs in some cases.

Interestingly, rheumatoid arthritis has for many years been linked with an excess of static electricity in the body, and when that is relieved there is often a lessening of the pain and discomfort. For this reason, many sufferers can be seen wearing a small copper wrist-bangle, which has the effect of 'earthing' the body. Similarly for many years, my late father recommended to patients that they walk barefoot on the lawn several times daily, and in many cases great relief was reported to him.

Medical practitioners often laugh at such methods, saying they are 'unproven' and 'quackery' – but in the absence of a safe 'modern' cure or treatment, such an attitude is really not called for. All treatments which can claim a success rate are deserving of study – and a copper bracelet has certainly never killed anyone – which is more than can be said for some recently prescribed chemical drugs!.

Herbal medicine has always concerned itself with a balanced treatment of an individual's ills, and it is for this reason that other aspects of the problem are looked at when a herbal practitioner makes recommendations.

With rheumatism and arthritis I have always found depression and mental tension to be serious side-effects, and effective treatment for them will often change patients' outlooks and allow them to face the future with more confidence. There are many safe herbal treatments available for tension, some of them shown in the herb section at the back of this book and others covered in a companion volume *Stress and Tension*.

Another noticeable side-effect is poor circulation. Here again, herbal treatment can be very effective and I would strongly recommend Vitamin E, and any herbal tablets containing Rutin.

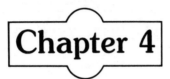

Chapter 4

The importance of diet

During consultations, I am often asked to give detailed diets. My answer to this is normally to suggest items best avoided for a particular illness, but to leave the actual details of the food to the patient's own good sense.

Putting it quite simply, if you suffer from a stomach ulcer and fried foods aggravate it, you should avoid them in the future. Similarly with most other illnesses, if certain food or drinks inflame and intensify the condition, then this is normally sufficient to act as a deterrent.

With rheumatism and arthritis, I have found from experience that there are certain foods and drinks which should not be taken regularly in the diet, since they can have an adverse effect. Mainly high acid content ones are the best to avoid. By this I mean citrus fruits and drinks (fresh orange, lemon, lime, grapefruit, rhubarb). Also, many greens, such as spring greens, Brussels sprouts and sometimes lettuce can have an adverse effect.

The main thing to avoid is a high concentration and, therefore, very occasional use will probably be of no harm. Generally speaking, a high protein diet should be avoided, particularly too much meat, and plenty of vegetables should be eaten. Following these simple diet suggestions can greatly help both conditions – and, of course, an avoidance of alcohol is also strongly recommended. Drink plenty of milk and eat small amounts regularly and often, avoiding very large meals.

Chapter 5

Herbal treatments and medication

The formulae in this chapter are all suitable to make at home following the given instructions and using quantities shown as percentages of the overall herb weight.

Ingredients should be available from herbalists and many health food shops – if any difficulty is experienced write direct to Cathay of Bournemouth Ltd, Cleveland Road, Bournemouth, BH1 4QG or consult the list of suppliers at the back of the book.

INFORMATION ON THE PREPARATION OF HERBS

DECOCTIONS

The herbs are cut, ground up or bruised and covered with cold fresh water. This mixture is then boiled for up to half an hour, allowed to cool and then strained through a fine mesh. Allow 28 grams of the herbs to 568 ml of water (1 oz to 1 pint). This method is normally used when the herb is unsuitable to make as an infusion. The usual dose is approximately one small wineglassful three times daily.

INFUSIONS

Tea is made by the process of infusion. Prepare the herbs to be used and quickly pour boiling water on them. Allow the mixture to stand for about half an hour, stirring frequently, and when ready strain off the liquid. Allow 28 grams to 568 ml of water (1 oz to 1 pint). The usual dose is approximately one small teacup or wineglassful three times daily; usually one after each main meal.

SOLID EXTRACTS
Start with a strong infusion of the herbs required and evaporate over low heat until a heavy consistency is obtained.

TINCTURES
This process is used for herbs and drugs which become useless when heated, or for those herbs which are not amenable to treatment by water. Tinctures are made with pure or diluted spirits of wine. Use 28 to 56 grams to 568 ml (1 to 2 oz to 1 pint). The dose varies according to strength of the main ingredient.

SOME SIMPLE FORMULAE TO MAKE AT HOME

A GOOD GENERAL HERB MIXTURE FOR RHEUMATISM
Oats (Avena)   2 parts
Dandelion Root   1 part
Paraguay Tea (Maté)   2 parts
Heather Flowers   1 part
Make up as an infusion.

A HERB MIXTURE FOR FIBROSITIS AND LUMBAGO
Sweet Chestnut   1 part
Devil's Claw   1 part
Make up as an infusion.

A HERB MIXTURE FOR MYALGIA

Buckbean	1 part
Wild Lettuce	1 part
Black Cohosh	1 part

Make up as an infusion.

A HERB MIXTURE FOR MUSCULAR RHEUMATISM

Wild Yam Root	1 part
Devil's Claw	1 part
Buckbean	1 part
Black Cohosh	1 part

Make up as an infusion.

A HERB MIXTURE FOR RHEUMATOID ARTHRITIS

Celery Seed	2 parts
Wintergreen	1 part
White Willow Bark	1 part
Wild Yam Root	1 part

Make up as an infusion.

AN ALTERNATIVE HERB MIXTURE FOR RHEUMATOID ARTHRITIS

Germander	1 part
Sarsparilla	1 part
White Poplar	1 part
Meadowsweet	1 part

Make up as an infusion.

A HERB MIXTURE FOR GOUT

Gravel Root	1 part
Germander	1 part
Pennyroyal	1 part
Guaiacum	1 part

Make up as a decoction.

A HERB MIXTURE FOR SCIATICA

Burdock Root	1 part
Buckbean	1 part
Wintergreen	1 part
St John's Wort	1 part

Make up as an infusion.

A GENERAL HERB POULTICE FOR EXTERNAL RHEUMATIC AND JOINT INFLAMMATION – ALSO HELPFUL FOR GOUT

Fenugreek Seeds	1 part
Savory Summer	2 parts
Capsicum	1 part
Marshmallow	2 parts
Mustard Seeds	1 part

Mix with hot water to make a comfortable warm poultice and loosely bind over affected area.

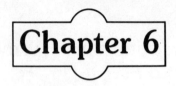

Chapter 6

Some recommended herbs

This section of the book lists in alphabetical order some of the herbs which can be used in the treatment of conditions mentioned earlier, together with other herbs of a generally beneficial nature.

A list of herbal suppliers will be given at the end of the section.

Mitton's Practical Modern Herbal, published by Foulsham, is recommended for a more complete list of medical herbs and their uses, together with much useful information.

ACACIA GUM (Acacia senegal)
Also known as   Gum Arabic.
Found wild   North Africa.
Appearance   Round tears obtained from spring shrub. Cuts are made in the bark and the gum exudes and coagulates.
Part used   Coagulated gum.
Therapeutic uses   An excellent demulcent, often used to relieve catarrh and chest complaints.
Prepared as   Mucilage by combining with hot water.

ADDER'S TONGUE, AMERICAN (Erythronium americanum)
Also known as   Snake's tongue.
Found wild   North America.
Appearance   Small bulbous plant with only two leaves; bright yellow lily-like flowers.
Part used   Leaves.

Therapeutic use   Generally as a poultice for ulcers and skin troubles.
Prepared as   Poultice.

AGAR-AGAR (Gilidium amansii)
Also known as   Japanese Isinglass.
Found wild   Japan.
Appearance   Prepared from a compound of several different seaweeds into thin strips of about 30 cm (12 ins) long from dried jelly.
Part used   Translucent strips.
Therapeutic use   Excellent for relief of stubborn constipation.
Prepared as   Powder.

AGRIMONY (Agrimonia eupatoria)
Also known as   Sticklewort.
Found wild   Throughout Northern Europe.
Appearance   A strong growing herb with green-grey leaves covered with soft hairs. Flowers are small and yellow on long slender spikes.
Part used   Herb.
Therapeutic uses   Dried leaves when infused make an astringent useful for diarrhoea; also as a tonic and diuretic.
Prepared as   Infusion.

ALDER, ENGLISH (Alnus glutinosa)
Found wild   England, Europe and North Africa.
Appearance   A small tree of distinctive appearance.
Parts used   Bark and leaves.
Therapeutic uses   The bark is used as a cathartic and the leaves to treat inflammation.
Prepared as   Decoction and poultice.

ALSTONIA BARK (Alstonia constricta)
Also known as   Fever Bark, Australian Quinine.
Found wild   Australia.

Appearance   Thick chocolate-coloured spongy bark from a moderate sized tree.
Part used   Bark.
Therapeutic uses   To prevent recurring bouts of malaria and for quick relief of most forms of rheumatism.
Prepared as   Powder or decoction.

AMARANTH (Amaranthus hypochondriacus)
Also known as   Love Lies Bleeding.
Found wild   UK and Europe.
Appearance   A common garden plant with crimson flowers similar to a coxcomb.
Part used   Herb.
Therapeutic uses   Treatment of diarrhoea and menorrhagia. As an astringent. Helpful in all cases of looseness of the bowel.
Prepared as   Decoction.

AMMONIACUM (Dorema Ammoniacum)
Also known as   Gum Ammoniacum.
Found wild   Turkey, Persia.
Appearance   Small rounded lumps, pale yellow in colour browning with age.
Part used   Gum resin.
Therapeutic uses   For respiratory troubles. Relief of catarrh, asthma, bronchitis.
Prepared as   Powder.

ANGELICA (Angelica archargelica)
Found wild   Europe, Asia.
Appearance   Plant growing from one and a half to two metres high.
Parts used   Root, seeds and herb.
Therapeutic uses   For rheumatic diseases, catarrh and asthma. A stimulant and diaphoretic.
Prepared as   Infusion or decoction.

ANISEED (Pimpinella anisum)

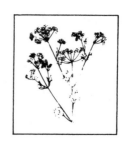

Found wild   Europe and North
Africa.
Appearance   An umbelliferous
plant with serrated leaves. Small
brownish-grey seeds.
Part used   Fruit.
Therapeutic use   A pectoral. Used
for cough medicines and elixirs.
Prepared as   Powder or decoction.

ARRACH (Chenopodium olidum)

Also known as   Goat's Arrach.
Found wild   Throughout Europe.
Appearance   A small inconspicuous herb with an
unpleasant odour.
Part used   Herb.
Therapeutic uses   As an emmenagogue to bring on
menstruation. Also an effective nervine.
Prepared as   Infusion.

AVENS (Geum urbanum)

Also known as   Colewort.
Found wild   Throughout Europe.
Appearance   Low-growing herb with yellow flowers.
Parts used   Herb and root.
Therapeutic uses   To stay bleeding and as a reliable tonic
for women. Also used for treating leucorrhea.
Prepared as   Decoction.

BALM OF GILEAD (Populus candicans)

Also known as   Several other plants are known as Balm
of Gilead.
Found wild   United States and Arabia.
Appearance   Strong gnarled shrub with feathery foliage.
Part used   Buds.

Therapeutic uses   Highly regarded as a tonic and diuretic. Excellent for chest troubles and rheumatic ailments.
Prepared as   Decoction or tincture.

BALMONY (Chelone glabra)
Also known as   Turtle Head, Snake Herb.
Found wild   United States and Canada.
Appearance   Low sturdy bush with oval dark leaves and white or pink flowers.
Part used   Leaves.
Therapeutic uses   Regarded as one of the best remedies for liver diseases. It is also antibilious, anthelmintic and a tonic.
Prepared as   Infusion.

BAYBERRY (Myrica cerifera)
Also known as   Waxberry, Candleberry.
Found wild   Europe and North America.
Appearance   A medium growing shrub with a profusion of large white berries.
Part used   Bark.
Therapeutic uses   A strong stimulant. A warming and effective deobstruent and cleanser. Also as a poultice for ulcers.
Prepared as   Infusion and poultice.

BEARSFOOT, AMERICAN (Polymnia uvedalia)
Also known as   Yellow Leaf Cup.
Found wild   North America.
Appearance   A tall branching plant found in rich loamy soil.
Part used   Root.
Therapeutic uses   Regarded as a valuable aid for quick pain relief, as a gentle laxative for the aged and as a stimulant.
Prepared as   Decoction.

BIRCH, EUROPEAN (Betula alba)

Found wild   Europe.
Appearance   A strikingly handsome tree common on gravel soils. Distinctive black and white bark.
Parts used   Bark and leaves.
Therapeutic uses   Birch tar oil makes a soothing ointment for skin disorders. The bark, as an infusion, is good for kidney stones.
Prepared as   Infusion and oil.

BISTORT (Polygonum bistorta)

Also known as   Adderwort.
Found wild   Europe and northern Britain.
Appearance   Low-growing herb chiefly found in ditches and damp places.
Part used   Root.
Therapeutic uses   Regarded as a cure for incontinence and as a gargle for sore throats.
Prepared as   Decoction.

BLACK ROOT (Leptandra virginica)

Also known as   Culver's Root.
Found wild   United States.
Appearance   A low-growing herb.
Part used   Rhizome.
Therapeutic uses   A blood purifying mixture. Also as a cathartic, diaphoretic and a liver stimulant.
Prepared as   Decoction.

BLADDERWRACK (Fucus vesiculosus)

Also known as   Seawrack or Kelpware.
Found wild   Around coasts of Britain.
Appearance   A large trailing dark green seaweed.
Part used   Dried plant.
Therapeutic uses   To help reduce obesity also to tone up the system and clear the kidneys.
Prepared as   Decoction.

BLUE FLAG (Iris versicolor)
Also known as   Flag Lily, Water Flag.
Where found   Extensively planted in gardens throughout Britain.
Appearance   A beautiful plant with arching strap-like leaves and blue, white, yellow or multi-colour flowers.
Part used   Rhizome.
Therapeutic uses   Principally as a blood purifier, also an alterative, diuretic and cathartic.
Prepared as   Decoction or powder.

BORAGE (Borago officinalis)
Also known as   Burrage.
Found wild   Throughout Europe.
Appearance   Bold, erect herb of strong growth. Small blue flowers.
Part used   Leaves.
Therapeutic uses   As a diuretic and demulcent and a flavouring agent.
Prepared as   Infusion and poultice.

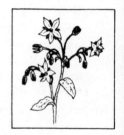

BOXWOOD, AMERICAN (Cornus florida)
Also known as   Dogwood, Cornel.
Found wild   United States.
Appearance   Small tree with rough bark and a profusion of pink spring flowers.
Parts used   Root and bark.
Therapeutic uses   As a tonic and stimulant also as a remedy for migraine and headaches.
Prepared as   Decoction or powder.

BROOM (Cytisus scoparius)
Also known as   Irish Broom.
Found wild   Throughout Europe.
Appearance   A small graceful arching shrub with profuse floral display.

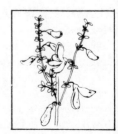

Part used   Top of each sprig.
Therapeutic uses   As a diuretic and cathartic. Also for relief of liver troubles and fluid retention.
Prepared as   Infusion.

BRYONY, BLACK (Tamus communis)
Found wild   Great Britain.
Appearance   An untidy climbing plant with alternate leaves.
Part used   Root.
Therapeutic uses   For the relief of rheumatic and arthritic pains and gout. An effective diuretic and a popular remedy for black eyes and bruises.
Prepared as   Poultice.

BRYONY, WHITE (Brionia dioica)
Found wild   Europe.
Appearance   Vine-like.
Part used   Root.
Therapeutic uses   Rheumatic pains, lumbago and gout. (Controlled dosage necessary.)
Prepared as   Decoction.

BUCHU (Barosma betulina)
Also known as   Bucco.
Found wild   Western coast of South Africa.
Appearance   Small procumbent herb growing in dry places.
Part used   Leaves.
Therapeutic uses   Urinary and bladder troubles. Also a diaphoretic and stimulant.
Prepared as   Infusion or decoction.

BUCKBEAN (Menyanthes trifoliata)
Also known as   Bogbean, Marsh Trefoil.
Found wild   UK and Europe.

Appearance   Aquatic plant.
Part used   Herb.
Therapeutic uses   Muscular rheumatism and rheumatoid arthritis.
Prepared as   Decoction.

BUGLOSS (Echium vulgare)

Also known as   Viper's Bugloss.
Found wild   Europe.
Appearance   A sturdy herb with blue flowers.
Part used   Herb.
Therapeutic uses   An expectorant and demulcent. Excellent for gentle bowel action. Also to clear phlegm from bronchial tubes.
Prepared as   Infusion.

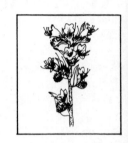

BURDOCK (Arctium lappa)

Also known as   Lappa.
Found wild   UK and Europe.
Appearance   Herb growing to as high as one and a half metres, with large rhubarb-shaped leaves.
Parts used   Herb, root and seeds.
Therapeutic uses   Rheumatism, gout, skin eruptions. Also a diuretic.
Prepared as   Decoction.

CAJAPUT (Melaleuca leucadendron)

Also known as   White Tea Tree.
Found wild   East Indies.
Appearance   A big bold tree.
Part used   Oil.
Therapeutic uses   For rheumatism and bruises. Also rubbed onto the gums for toothache. Taken on sugar to end hiccoughs.
Prepared as   Oil.

CANELLA (Canella alba)

Also known as   Wild Cinnamon.
Found wild   West Indies.
Appearance   Slender branching tree with light grey bark.
Part used   Bark.
Therapeutic uses   Stimulant tonic for the aged. Promotes digestion and elimination and prevents flatulence.
Prepared as   Decoction.

CAPSICUM (Capsicum minimum)

Also known as   Cayenne, Chillies.
Found wild   Tropical countries including Africa and South America.
Appearance   Small shrub with red fruits.
Part used   Fruit.
Therapeutic uses   An aid to the digestive system. Tonic. As an external lotion for lumbago.
Prepared as   Powder.

CAROBA (Jacaranda procera)

Also known as   Carob Tree.
Found wild   South Africa and South America.
Appearance   A handsome tree with lanceolate leaves.
Part used   Leaves.
Therapeutic uses   As a diaphoretic and diuretic. Also a safe sedative.
Prepared as   Infusion.

CASCARILLA (Croton eleuteria)

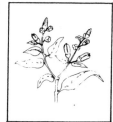

Also known as   Sweet Wood Bark.
Found wild   The Bahamas and West Indies.
Appearance   A diminutive tree.
Part used   Bark.
Therapeutic use   A tonic stimulant.
Prepared as   Decoction.

CATNIP (Nepeta cataria)
Also known as   Catmint.
Found wild   Britain.
Appearance   A procumbent grey plant.
Part used   Herb.
Therapeutic uses   Carminative and diaphoretic and has tonic properties. Also used for the relief of piles.
Prepared as   Infusion.

CAYENNE, HUNGARIAN (Capsicum tetragonum)
Also known as   Paprika.
Found wild   Hungary, also cultivated elsewhere.
Appearance   A strong growing herb with large green fruits.
Part used   Fruit.
Therapeutic use   Rich source of vitamin C.
Prepared as   Powder.

CELERY (Apium graveolens)
Found wild   Europe.
Appearance   This is the familiar vegetable.
Parts used   Stem and seeds.
Therapeutic uses   A tonic diuretic and carminative and an aid for rheumatoid troubles. Also regarded as an effective aphrodisiac.
Prepared as   Decoction or powder from the seeds.

CHAMOMILE, BELGIAN (Anthemis nobilis)
Found wild   Belgium and France. Widely cultivated.
Appearance   Herb with double flowers.
Part used   Flowers.
Therapeutic uses   Widely used for women suffering from nervous upsets and as a tonic, stomachic and antispasmodic.
Prepared as   Infusion.

CHAMOMILE, GERMAN (Matricaria chamomilla)

Found wild   Europe.
Appearance   Herb with small cushion-like flowers in profusion.
Part used   Flowers.
Therapeutic uses   Excellent nerve sedative, carminative and tonic.
Prepared as   Infusion.

CHICKWEED (Stellaria media)

Also known as   Starweed.
Found wild   Britain.
Appearance   Small prolific weed.
Part used   Herb.
Therapeutic uses   A demulcent and to allay feverish conditions.
Prepared as   Decoction.

CHIRETTA (Swertia chirata)

Also known as   Indian Gentian.
Found wild   India.
Appearance   Small wiry herb growing in arid places.
Part used   Herb.
Therapeutic use   Tonic to restore flagging appetite.
Prepared as   Decoction.

CLUBMOSS (Lycopodium clavatum)

Found wild   Northern hemisphere.
Appearance   Low spreading greyish-green plant usually found near water.
Part used   Herb.
Therapeutic uses   Treatment of cystitis, kidney complaints and urinary disorders. Also a sedative and for stomach disorders.
Prepared as   Infusion.

COHOSH, BLACK (Cimicifuga racemosa)
Also known as   Bugbane.
Found wild   North America.
Appearance   Herb.
Part used   Rhizome.
Therapeutic uses   Rheumatic complaints, astringent, emmenagogue.
Prepared as   Decoction.

COHOSH, BLUE (Caulophyllum thalictroides)
Also known as   Blueberry Root.
Found wild   United States and Canada.
Appearance   A gnarled, crowded shrub.
Part used   Rhizome.
Therapeutic uses   As a diuretic and emmenagogue and also as a vermifuge to expel worms. Aids rheumatic sufferers and women's complaints.
Prepared as   Decoction.

COMFREY (Symphytum officinale)
Also known as   Knitbone, Slippery Root.
Found wild   Throughout the UK and Europe.
Appearance   Fleshy-leaved plant which can grow to approximately one metre.
Parts used   Leaves and root.
Therapeutic uses   Helpful for treatment of internal ulcers. For rheumatic pains and for arthritis, and a poultice for treatment of bruises and sprains.
Prepared as   Decoction.

CONDURANGO (Marsdenia condurango)
Found wild   South America.
Appearance   Climbing vine found in heavily forested areas.
Part used   Bark.
Therapeutic uses   An alterative and stomachic. Helpful for treating duodenal ulcers.
Prepared as   Decoction.

CORNSILK (Zea mays)
Found wild   South Africa and America.
Appearance   Maize.
Part used   Part of flower.·
Therapeutic uses   Principally as a diuretic but also for pulmonary troubles.
Prepared as   Decoction.

COTTON ROOT (Gossypium herbaceum)
Found wild   Mediterranean islands and United States.
Appearance   Twists of bark.
Part used   Bark of root.
Therapeutic uses   Treatment of women's disorders.
Prepared as   Infusion and oil.

COUCHGRASS (Agropyron repens)
Also known as   Twitchgrass.
Found wild   In most parts of the world.
Appearance   A strong grass with white fleshy roots.
Part used   Rhizome.
Therapeutic uses   For treatment of cystitis, nephritis and bladder troubles. Also for rheumatoid ills and as a diuretic and aperient.
Prepared as   Infusion.

CRAMP BARK (Viburnum opulus)
Also known as   Snow-ball Tree, Guelder Rose.
Found wild   Europe and America.
Appearance   Strong-growing bush with white ball-shaped flowers.
Part used   Bark.
Therapeutic uses   As a nervine for treatment of spasms and convulsions. Antispasmodic. A safe children's medication.
Prepared as   Decoction.

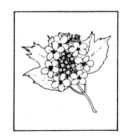

CRANESBILL, AMERICAN (Geranium maculatum)

Also known as   Wild Geranium, Storksbill.
Found wild   United States.
Appearance   Shrubby small herb with blue flowers.
Parts used   Herb and root.
Therapeutic uses   Has quick styptic properties and is a tonic and astringent. Treatment for piles and ulcers.
Prepared as   Decoction.

DAMIANA (Turnera diffusa)

Found wild   Southern United States and Mexico.
Appearance   Medium-sized shrub.
Parts used   Leaves and stem.
Therapeutic uses   Famous for its aphrodisiac qualities. As a tonic safe for the aged and those suffering from exhaustion and debility.
Prepared as   Infusion.

DANDELION (Taraxacus officinale)

Found wild   Most temperate climates.
Appearance   Common herb with long root, toothed leaves and bright yellow flowers.
Parts used   Leaves and root.
Therapeutic uses   As a tonic and diuretic and for liver and kidney ills. Roots frequently used for coffee as it contains no caffeine.
Prepared as   Infusion or decoction.

DEVIL'S CLAW (Harpagophytum procumbens)

Found wild   Southern part of Africa.
Appearance   Low-growing plant.
Part used   Root.
Therapeutic uses   Of great value for the treatment of inflammatory and rheumatic conditions. Also has sedative and diuretic properties.
Prepared as   Decoction.

DOG ROSE (Rosa canina)

Also known as   Wild Briar.
Found wild   Europe and the Middle East.
Appearance   The wild rambling rose.
Part used   Fruit.
Therapeutic uses   The fruit yields ascorbic acid (vitamin C) of great value when given to young children.
Prepared as   Syrup.

ECHINACEA (Echinacea angustifolia)

Also known as   Coneflower.
Found wild   United States.
Appearance   Herb of medium height.
Part used   Rhizome.
Therapeutic uses   As an antiseptic and alterative and to help purify the blood. Also for typhoid.
Prepared as   Decoction.

ELDER (Sambucus nigra)

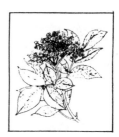

Also known as   Black Elder.
Found wild   Europe.
Appearance   A tall straggling shrub with profuse crops of black berries.
Parts used   Flowers, berries and bark.
Therapeutic uses   For colds and influenza. As an alterative and diuretic. It is a safe soporific and induces healthy sleep.
Prepared as   Infusion.

EVENING PRIMROSE (Oenothera biennis)

Also known as   Tree Primrose.
Found wild   European gardens.

Appearance   A small herb with a delightful display of yellow flowers.
Parts used   Leaves and bark.
Therapeutic uses   As a sedative and astringent. For the relief of menstrual disorders.
Prepared as   Decoction.

FENUGREEK (Trigonella foenum-graecum)

Found wild   Mediterranean area, North Africa and India.
Appearance   Slender stemmed plant.
Part used   Herb.
Therapeutic uses   As an emolient, a laxative and expectorant. Can be applied externally to assist gout.
Prepared as   Decoction and poultice.

FEVERFEW (Chrysanthemum parthenium)

Also known as   Featherfew.
Found wild   Throughout Europe.
Appearance   A small grey herb with hairy stems.
Part used   Herb.

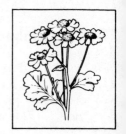

Therapeutic uses   As an aperient, also used by women to bring on the menses. Now recognised as an aid to migraine.
Prepared as   Infusion.

FIGWORT (Scrophularia nodosa)

Also known as   Throatwort.
Found wild   Throughout Europe.
Appearance   Medium-sized tree of rampant growth.
Part used   Herb.
Therapeutic uses   Aperient also an emollient and demulcent and as a poultice for ulcers.
Prepared as   Infusion and poultice.

FRINGETREE (Chionanthus virginica)

Found wild   Southern United States.

Appearance   A small tree with inconspicuous white flowers. It has a very bitter taste.

Part used   The bark of the root.

Therapeutic uses   Tonic, alterative and diuretic. Also used for the treatment of liver disorders, gallstones and jaundice.

Prepared as   Decoction.

GARLIC (Allium sativum)

Where found   Universally cultivated.

Appearance   Similar to a shallot.

Part used   Bulb.

Therapeutic uses   For treatment of dyspepsia and flatulence, also as a stimulant.

Prepared as   Juice and tincture.

GENTIAN (Gentiana lutea)

Found wild   Alpine meadows.

Appearance   A plant with oblong, pale-green leaves and large, yellow, scented flowers.

Part used   Root.

Therapeutic use   Tonic.

Prepared as   Decoction or powder.

GERMANDER (Teucrium chamaedrys)

Also known as   Wall Germander.

Found wild   UK and Europe.

Appearance   Stemmed plant growing to about half a metre.

Part used   Herb.

Therapeutic uses   A helpful plant for the treatment of rheumatoid arthritis and gout. Has anti-inflammatory properties.

Prepared as   Decoction.

GINGER (Zingiber officinale)

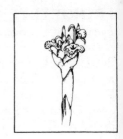

Found wild   West Indies and China.
Appearance   About one metre high with glossy aromatic leaves.
Part used   Rhizome.
Therapeutic uses   Has stimulative and carminative properties and can be used as an expectorant and an aid to digestion.
Prepared as   Powder or decoction.

GINSENG (Panax quinquefolium)

Also known as   Chinese Panacea, Panax.
Found wild   China and Mongolia.
Appearance   Erect-growing herb with vivid fleshy leaves.
Part used   Root.
Therapeutic uses   An effective aphrodisiac and tonic. Also aids digestive problems.
Prepared as   Powder or decoction.

GOLDEN SEAL (Hydrastis canadensis)

Also known as   Yellow Root.
Where found   Cultivated in North America.
Appearance   Tall growing herb with disagreeable odour.
Part used   Rhizome.
Therapeutic uses   For gastric disorders and as a soothing laxative and tonic.
Prepared as   Decoction or powder.

GOUTWORT (Aegopodium podagraria)

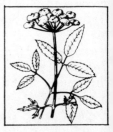

Also known as   Goutweed.
Found wild   Throughout Europe.
Appearance   A small spreading herb.

Part used   Herb.
Therapeutic uses   As a sedative and diuretic. For the relief of sciatica and gout and of value when used as a poultice.
Prepared as   Decoction and poultice.

GRAVEL ROOT (Eupatorium purpureum)

Also known as   Gravel Weed.
Found wild   North America.
Appearance   Herb growing to about a metre high.
Part used   Rhizome.
Therapeutic uses   Diuretic and anti-rheumatic. Helpful in cases of gout, rheumatism, kidney stones and cystitis.
Prepared as   Decoction.

GUAIACUM (Guaiacum officinale)

Also known as   Lignum Vitae.
Found wild   West Indies and South America.
Appearance   A strong tree producing the strongest wood in the world.

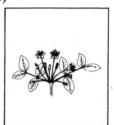

Parts used   Wood and resin.
Therapeutic uses   For the relief of rheumatism, and as a diaphoretic and alterative.
Prepared as   Decoction.

GUARANA (Paulinia cupana)

Also known as   Brazilian Cocoa.
Found wild   Brazil.
Appearance   A tall arching shrub.
Part used   Seeds.
Therapeutic uses   As a stimulant and for relief of headaches and migraine. Also used by women to bring on menses and effective in treatment of arthritis.
Prepared as   Decoction or powder.

HAWTHORN (Crataegus oxycantha)

Also known as   May Tree.
Found wild   Throughout Britain.
Appearance   A common small tree.
Part used   Fruit.
Therapeutic uses   As an aid for heart conditions.
Prepared as   Decoction.

HEATHER FLOWERS (Calluna vulgaris)

Also known as   Ling Flowers.
Found wild   UK and Europe.
Appearance   Evergreen shrub.
Part used   Flowers.
Therapeutic uses   Has anti-rheumatic properties and is also a diuretic. Has proved useful in cases of cystitis, gout and rheumatic pains.
Prepared as   Infusion.

HOLLY (Ilex aquifolium)

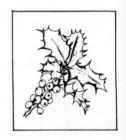

Found wild   Throughout Europe.
Appearance   A small tree with glossy, shiny leaves with a profusion of red or yellow berries in winter.
Part used   Fruit.
Therapeutic uses   Mostly to relieve chest trouble and laryngitis.
Prepared as   Decoction.

HOPS (Humulus lupulus)

Found wild   Europe, and cultivated in most parts of the world.
Appearance   A climbing vine.
Part used   Flowers.
Therapeutic uses   As an anodyne for the relief of pain. Also as a tonic and an aid for stomach disorders and to promote sleep.
Prepared as   Infusion.

HORSERADISH (Cochlearia armoracia)

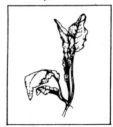

Found wild   Europe.
Appearance   A herb growing to one metre with a pungent odour.
Part used   Root.
Therapeutic uses   Relieves flatulence and indigestion. Promotes perspiration and is a diuretic.
Prepared as   Infusion.

HORSETAIL (Equisetum arvense)

Also known as   Scouring Rushes.
Found wild   Britain.
Appearance   A tall bold herb with cane-like appearance.
Part used   Herb.
Therapeutic uses   A powerful astringent and also a diuretic. Excellent for kidney troubles.
Prepared as   Decoction.

HOUNDSTONGUE (Cynoglossum officinale)

Found wild   Britain.
Appearance   A medium-sized herb with long, strap-like leaves.
Part used   Herb.
Therapeutic uses   An anodyne for quick relief of pain. Also as a demulcent for soothing coughs and colds. Can also be used to reduce piles.
Prepared as   Infusion.

HOUSELEEK (Sempervivum tectorum)

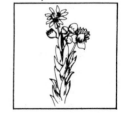

Found wild   Throughout Britain.
Appearance   Small procumbent plant.
Part used   Leaves.
Therapeutic uses   As an astringent and poultice. Commonly used to soften corns and hard skin.
Prepared as   Infusion.

HYDROCOTYLE (Hydrocotyle asiatica)
Also known as   Indian Pennywort.
Found wild   Tropical India and Africa.
Appearance   A small plant similar to Angelica.
Part used   Leaves.
Therapeutic uses   As an aphrodisiac and also useful for treatment of urinary disorders.
Prepared as   Infusion.

ICELAND MOSS (Cetraria islandica)
Found wild   Throughout the northern hemisphere.
Appearance   This is not a moss but a procumbent grey lichen.
Part used   Plant.
Therapeutic uses   For catarrh and bronchitis. It is a nutritive and helpful for digestive complaints.
Prepared as   Decoction.

JABORANDI (Pilocarpus microphyllus)
Found wild   Brazil.
Appearance   A small herb.
Part used   Leaves.
Therapeutic uses   A diaphoretic and expectorant and is beneficial to asthma sufferers.
Prepared as   Infusion.

JALAP (Ipomaega purga)
Found wild   South America.
Appearance   A robust climbing plant.
Part used   Root.
Therapeutic use   As a purgative.
Prepared as   Decoction.

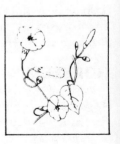

JAMBUL (Eugenia jambolana)
Also known as   Java Plum.
Found wild   East India.
Appearance   A large spreading tree.

Part used   Seeds.
Therapeutic uses   Helpful to diabetics. Quickly reduces urinal sugar content.
Prepared as   Decoetion.

KAVA (Piper methysticum)
Also known as   Kava-Kava.
Found wild   South Pacific.
Appearance   Tall shrub.
Part used   Root.
Therapeutic uses   As a tonic and as a diuretic. Helpful for the treatment of joint pains, rheumatism and gout.
Prepared as   Decoction.

KUMARHOU (Pomaderris elliptica)
Found wild   North Island of New Zealand.
Appearance   A very pretty shrub.
Part used   Herb.
Therapeutic uses   As a panacea and for the treatment of rheumatism and pulmonary disorders. Also as a blood purifier.
Prepared as   Infusion.

LAUREL (Laurus nobilis)
Also known as   Bay Tree.
Found wild   Europe.
Appearance   An evergreen tree with lanceolate leaves which grows up to seven or eight metres high.
Parts used   Leaves, fruit and oil.
Therapeutic uses   As a stomachic and the oil is used as a relief for rheumatism.
Prepared as   Oil for external application.

LETTUCE, WILD (Lactuca virosa)
Found wild   Warm parts of Europe.
Appearance   A small plant of bushy appearance.
Parts used   Leaves and juice.

Therapeutic uses   An anodyne and sedative. Also useful
to ease coughs of nervous origin. Relieves rheumatic pain.
Prepared as   Decoction.

LIME FLOWERS (Tilia europoea)

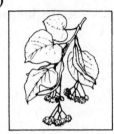

Also known as   Linden Flowers.
Found wild   Throughout Europe.
Appearance   A graceful tree.
Part used   Flowers.
Therapeutic uses   A strong but safe
nervine for relief of headaches and
hysteria. Stimulant and tonic.
Prepared as   Infusion.

LIQUORICE (Glycyrrhiza glabra)

Found wild   Europe and Middle East.
Appearance   A strong-growing perennial plant.
Part used   Root.
Therapeutic uses   In cough medicines. As a demulcent
and pectoral and as a gentle laxative.
Prepared as   Decoction.

LOBELIA (Lobelia inflata)

Found wild   United States.
Appearance   A small trailing herb.
Part used   Herb.
Therapeutic uses   As a stimulant, diaphoretic and
expectorant.
Prepared as   Infusion.

LOGWOOD (Haematoxylon campechianum)

Found wild   South America.
Appearance   A massive tree.
Part used   Wood.
Therapeutic uses   To relieve diarrhoea and dysentery.
Also helpful for women's disorders.
Prepared as   Decoction.

MANACA (Brunfelsia hopeana)
Found wild   South America and West Indies.
Appearance   A spindly shrub.
Part used   Root.
Therapeutic uses   An alterative and for the treatment of arthritis.
Prepared as   Decoction.

MANNA (Fraxinus ornus)
Found wild   Mediterranean countries.
Appearance   Medium-sized shrub.
Part used   Sap from cuts in bark.
Therapeutic uses   As a gentle laxative for pregnant women and as a nutritive invalid food.
Prepared as   Decoction.

MARSHMALLOW (Althaea officinalis)
Found wild   Throughout Europe.
Appearance   A strong-growing herb usually found in watery places.
Parts used   Leaves and root.
Therapeutic uses   As an emollient and demulcent for incorporation in cough medicines. Also for treatment of cystitis and for soothing the alimentary canal.
Prepared as   Infusion and poultice.

MAYWEED (Anthemis cotula)
Also known as   Dog Fennel.
Found wild   Throughout Europe.
Appearance   A low-growing herb and common weed.
Part used   Herb.
Therapeutic uses   An antispasmodic with marked tonic qualities. Excellent for migraine.
Prepared as   Infusion.

MEADOWSWEET (Filipendula ulmaria)
Also known as   Bridewort.

Found wild   UK and Europe.
Appearance   Long-stemmed herb
growing to almost one metre.
Part used   Herb.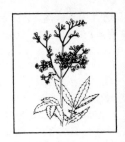
Therapeutic uses   Anti-rheumatic,
stomachic, astringent. Helpful for
severe cases of cystitis. Muscular,
rheumatic and joint pains.
Prepared as   Infusion.

MEZEREON (Daphne mesereum)
Also known as   Spurge Laurel.
Found wild   Europe.
Appearance   A strong crowded shrub.
Parts used   Bark and root.
Therapeutic uses   A stimulant. For relief of rheumatism.
Prepared as   Decoction.

MOTHERWORT (Leonurus cardiaca)
Where found   A common garden plant in Britain and
northern Europe.
Appearance   A pink flowered shrub of handsome
appearance.
Part used   Herb.
Therapeutic uses   A nervine and for the relief of women's
troubles. Also a tonic and stimulant and helpful for heart
conditions.
Prepared as   Infusion.

MULLEIN (Verbascum thapsus)
Found wild   Throughout Europe.
Appearance   Tall perennial cylindrical plant with a
tower of yellow flowers.
Parts used   Leaves and flowers.
Therapeutic uses   For lung and bronchial inflammations.
As an astringent, demulcent and pectoral.
Prepared as   Infusion.

MUSTARD, BLACK (Brassica nigra)
MUSTARD, WHITE (Brassica alba)
Found wild   Throughout the northern hemisphere.
Appearance   A short-growing annual herb with bright yellow flowers.
Part used   Seeds.
Therapeutic uses   A powerful irritant and emetic. For relief of rheumatic and arthritic pain.
Prepared as   Poultice.

MYRTLE (Myrtus communis)
Found wild   The warmer areas of Europe.
Appearance   A strong bushy shrub.
Part used   Leaves.
Therapeutic uses   Often used as a balm for night cramp.
Prepared as   Infusion and poultice.

NIGHT BLOOMING CEREUS (Cereus grandiflorus)
Found wild   Jamaica.
Appearance   A small branded cactus with large creamy flowers.
Part used   Plant.
Therapeutic uses   An effective heart stimulant and for relief of palpitations. Also a diuretic and helpful for prostate diseases.
Prepared as   Decoction.

NUTMEG (Myristica fragrans)
Found wild   Malaysia, Indonesia and the West Indies.
Appearance   Tall tree.
Parts used   Seeds and oil.
Therapeutic uses   Carminative, anti-emetic. Helpful in most cases of stomach upset. Can be used externally for the treatment of rheumatic pain. Use nutmeg in moderation.
Prepared as   Powder and oil.

OATS (Avena sativa)
Found wild   In most temperate climates.
Appearance   A common farm crop similar to wheat.
Part used   Seeds.
Therapeutic uses   An effective nerve tonic and to allay spasms. Relieves rheumatic pain.
Prepared as   Decoction.

PAPAW (Carica papaya)
Also known as   Melon Tree.
Found wild   Throughout sub-tropical areas.
Appearance   A tall tree (about seven metres) with boldly serated leaves. Only the female produces fruit.
Part used   Papain from the juice.
Therapeutic uses   As a digestive aid, helpful for duodenal and peptic ulcers.
Prepared as   Powder.

PARAGUAY TEA (Ilex paraguensis)
Also known as   Mate Tea.
Found wild   South America.
Appearance   A dense shrub.
Part used   Leaves.
Therapeutic uses   Stimulant. Very helpful in the relief of rheumatism and arthritis. Commonly used to make a pleasant tea.
Prepared as   Infusion.

PARSLEY (Carum petroselinum)
Found wild   Europe.
Appearance   Bienniel umbelliferous plant with white flowers and aromatic leaves.
Parts used   Seeds, root and leaves.
Therapeutic uses   As a diuretic and in the treatment of kidney disorders, stones and gravel. Emmenagogue and in the treatment of amenorrhoea.
Prepared as   Decoction.

PARSLEY PIERT (Alchemilla arvensis)

Also known as   Beakstone.
Found wild   Throughout Europe.
Appearance   A low-growing herb
with tiny green flowers. Not related
to common parsley.
Part used   Herb.
Therapeutic uses   For the relief of
bladder and kidney troubles and
helpful in dissolving kidney stones.
Prepared as   Infusion.

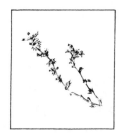

PARSLEY ROOT (Petroselinum crispum)

Found wild   UK and Europe.
Appearance   Small herb.
Part used   Root.
Therapeutic use   Carminative, diuretic, emmenagogue.
Has useful anti-rheumatic properties.
Prepared as   Decoction.

PENNYROYAL (Mentha pulegium)

Found wild   UK and Europe.
Appearance   Low-growing herb.
Parts used   Herb and oil.
Therapeutic uses   Carminative, emmenagogue,
stimulant, diaphoretic. This herb has always been regarded
as a reliable treatment for obstructed menstruation.
Applied externally it is helpful for gout.
Prepared as   Infusion.

PEONY (Paeonia officinalis)

Found wild   Southern Asia.
Appearance   Beautiful perennial that bears vivid double
flowers in profusion.
Part used   Root.
Therapeutic uses   Antispasmodic and tonic.
Prepared as   Infusion.

PEPPERMINT (Mentha piperita)
Also known as   Curled Mint.
Found wild   Europe and North America.
Appearance   A stately herb with purple-hued stems.
Part used   Herb.
Therapeutic uses   Stomachic and carminative. Relieves sickness, flatulence and indigestion.
Prepared as   Infusion.

PICHI (Fabiana imbricata)
Found wild   South America.
Appearance   Herb of moderate growth with tiny leaves.
Parts used   Leaves and wood.
Therapeutic uses   Hepatic. Recommended for treatment of liver disorders. Also a stimulant and diuretic and helpful for catarrhal and kidney troubles.
Prepared as   Infusion.

PIPSISSIWA (Chimaphila umbellata)
Also known as   Ground Holly.
Found wild   Northern hemisphere.
Appearance   A small tough shrub.
Part used   Leaves.
Therapeutic uses   As a tonic and alterative. Helpful for rheumatoid ailments.
Prepared as   Infusion.

POKE ROOT (Phytolacca decandra)
Found wild   North America.
Appearance   Shrub with multitude of grape-sized black berries.
Parts used   Root and berries.
Therapeutic uses   For relief of rheumatism and arthritis. Also an emetic and cathartic.
Prepared as   Decoction.

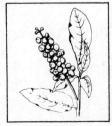

POPLAR, WHITE (Populus tremuloides)

Found wild   UK and Europe.
Appearance   Large tree.
Part used   Bark.
Therapeutic uses   Anti-rheumatic.
Anti-inflammatory, antiseptic.
Beneficial in all cases of muscular and
arthritic rheumatism.
Prepared as   Decoction.

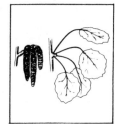

PRICKLY ASH (Zanthoxylum clavaherculis)

Found wild   North America.
Appearance   Medium-sized tree.
Parts used   Bark and berries.
Therapeutic uses   Diaphoretic, carminative, stimulant.
Helpful for circulation disorders associated with
rheumatism.
Prepared as   Decoction.

QUASSIA (Picraena excelsa)

Found wild   West Indies.
Appearance   A tree of great stature.
Part used   Wood.
Therapeutic uses   As a tonic and also effective for
treatment of stomach disorders. Helpful for cramp.
Prepared as   Infusion.

RAGWORT (Senecio jacobaea)

Also known as   St James's Wort.
Found wild   Throughout Europe.
Appearance   Erect slender herb with yellow flower.
Part used   Herb.
Therapeutic uses   For rheumatic conditions and gout.
Also helpful for lung and bronchial infections and can
be applied as an ointment.
Prepared as   Decoction and poultice.

RED SAGE (Salvia officinalis)

Also known as   Sage.
Found wild   Europe and North America.
Appearance   A small herb.
Part used   Leaves.
Therapeutic uses   An astringent, helpful for sore throats, quinsy and laryngitis.
Prepared as   Infusion.

REST HARROW (Omonis spinosa)

Found wild   Throughout Britain.
Appearance   A common herb about 60 cm high. Prickly, with small purple flowers.
Part used   Root.
Therapeutic uses   Diuretic. Helpful for rheumatism.
Prepared as   Infusion.

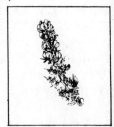

ST JOHN'S WORT (Hypericum perforatum)

Found wild   Britain.
Appearance   Sturdy yellow-flowered herb.
Part used   Herb.
Therapeutic uses   Diuretic. Expectorant, helpful for coughs and bronchial ailments.
Prepared as   Decoction.

SAMPHIRE (Crithmum maritimum)

Also known as   Rock Samphire.
Found wild   England, particularly in saline conditions.
Appearance   A small herb that prefers shelter of rocks.
Part used   Herb.
Therapeutic uses   Diuretic with a beneficial kidney action. Helpful for weight loss.
Prepared as   Infusion.

SARSPARILLA (Smilax medica)
Found wild   South America.
Appearance   Bush.
Part used   Rhizome.
Therapeutic uses   Alterative, anti-
rheumatic, antiseptic. Helpful in
cases of psoriasis and other skin
ailments. Long-standing treatment
for severe rheumatism and
rheumatoid arthritis.
Prepared as   Decoction.

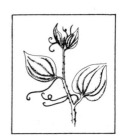

SASSAFRAS (Sassafras variifolium)
Found wild   Pacific coast of North America.
Appearance   A shrub of average size found in
mountainous regions.
Parts used   Bark and root.
Therapeutic uses   Strong stimulant and often used as an
aphrodisiac. Also effective for arthritis and rheumatism.
Prepared as   Infusion.

SAVORY, SUMMER (Satureia hortensis)
Where found   Commonly cultivated throughout the
world.
Appearance   A small shrubby plant.
Part used   Herb.
Therapeutic uses   For relief of flatulence and indigestion.
Also as a poultice to reduce inflammations.
Prepared as   Decoction and poultice.

SENNA (Cassia angustifolia)
Found wild   Arabia.
Appearance   Tree of sparse growth with distinctive grey-
green leaves.
Parts used   Leaves and seed case.
Therapeutic uses   A safe laxative without purging effect.
Prepared as   Infusion.

SHEPHERD'S PURSE (Capsella bursa-pastoris)
Found wild   Everywhere.
Appearance   Small insignificant weed with little white flowers.
Part used   Herb.
Therapeutic uses   Diuretic, usually for kidney and urinary troubles. Antiscorbutic, prevents scurvy.
Prepared as   Infusion.

SLIPPERY ELM (Ulmus fulva)
Found wild   North America.
Appearance   A great tree of spreading growth.
Part used   Inner part of bark.
Therapeutic uses   As a nutritive for invalids. Also an emollient and demulcent for healing burns and skin troubles.
Prepared as   Infusion or powder.

SPEARMINT (Mentha viridis)
Found wild   Throughout the northern hemisphere.
Appearance   Strong-growing perennial herb.
Therapeutic uses   Stimulant. Carminative. Suitable for the very young and old.
Prepared as   Infusion.

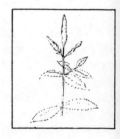

SQUILL (Urfinea maritima)
Found wild   Southern Europe and North Africa.
Appearance   One of the lily family.
Part used   Corm.
Therapeutic uses   Expectorant. Helpful in relieving catarrh, asthma and bronchial troubles. Also a cathartic and diuretic.
Prepared as   Decoction.

SWAMP MILKWEED (Asclepias incarnata)

Found wild   United States.
Appearance   Medium-sized shrub of grotesque appearance.
Part used   Rhizome and root.
Therapeutic uses   Cathartic. Emetic. Beneficial in treatment of arthritis and stomach disorders.
Prepared as   Infusion.

SWEET CHESTNUT (Castanea sativa)

Found wild   UK and Europe.
Appearance   Large tree.
Part used   Leaves.
Therapeutic uses   Astringent. Anti-rheumatic. Helpful in cases of muscular rheumatism, lumbago and fibrositis. Of specific benefit to catarrhal conditions.
Prepared as   Infusion.

WATER BETONY (Scrophularia aquatica)

Found wild   United States.
Appearance   Medium-sized herb that grows beside water.
Part used   Leaves.
Therapeutic uses   Used as an ointment and poultices for skin complaints. An excellent vulnerary.
Prepared as   Poultice.

WATER DOCK (Rumex aquaticus)

Also known as   Bloodwort.
Found wild   Throughout Europe.
Appearance   One of the common dock family.
Part used   Root.
Therapeutic uses   An alterative and detergent. Helps clean and strengthen gums and relieves mouth ulcers.
Prepared as   Infusion or powder.

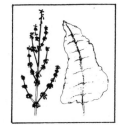

WILD CARROT (Caucus carota)

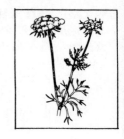

Found wild   UK and Europe.
Appearance   Small version of
cultivated carrot.
Part used   Herb.
Therapeutic uses   Diuretic,
carminative. Helpful in cases of
cystitis, bladder infection and gout.
Prepared as   Infusion.

WILD YAM ROOT (Dioscorea villosa)

Also known as   Rheumatism Root, Colic Root.
Found wild   North America and tropical areas.
Appearance   Tuberous plant.
Part used   Root.
Therapeutic uses   Anti-inflammatory, antispasmodic,
diaphoretic. Helpful in the treatment of rheumatoid
arthritis and muscular rheumatism. Leg cramps and
intermittent claudication are two other conditions which
can be beneficially treated.
Prepared as   Decoction.

WILLOW, WHITE (Salix alba)

Also known as   Common Willow.
Found wild   Europe.
Appearance   Tree that grows by
streams and rivers.

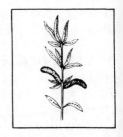

Parts used   Bark and leaves.
Therapeutic uses   A tonic that
relieves rheumatic and arthritic
conditions. Also an anti-periodic.
Prepared as   Decoction.

WINTERGREEN (Gaultheria procumbens)

Found wild   North America.
Appearance   A small procumbent shrub.
Part used   Leaves.

Therapeutic uses   As an astringent that controls diarrhoea. Stimulant. Used as a remedy for rheumatism and as an embrocation.
Prepared as   Infusion and ointment.

WOOD SAGE (Teucrium scorodonia)
Also known as   Garlic Sage.
Found wild   UK.
Appearance   Small herb.
Part used   Herb.
Therapeutic uses   Respiratory infections. Astringent, anti-rheumatic. This herb has been used for many years to treat respiratory infections and also rheumatic pain and stiffness.
Prepared as   infusion

YARROW (Achillea millefolium)
Also known as   Milfoil.
Found wild   Britain.
Appearance   A tiny herb.
Part used   Herb.
Therapeutic uses   A stimulant and diaphoretic. Excellent for treatment of influenza and heavy chest colds. Helpful for blood purifying.
Prepared as   Infusion.

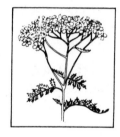

A guide to herbal suppliers

Herbalists tend to be rather thin on the ground and while your local Health Food Shop should be able to assist with the more common dried herbs, specialist requirements often need specialist stockists.

The following list is by no means a complete one, but should be sufficient to cover most herbs mentioned in the book.

MAIL ORDER STOCKISTS

Cathay of Bournemouth Ltd
Cleveland Road
Bournemouth
BH1 4QG.
(Free literature on request)

Culpeper Ltd
Handstock Road
Linton
Cambs
CB1 6NJ

MAJOR RETAIL OUTLETS

Bournemouth
Cathay of Bournemouth Ltd
Cleveland Road
Bournemouth
and
Hampshire House
Bourne Avenue
Central Bournemouth

Gerard House
736 Christchurch Road
Bournemouth
and
31 St Thomas Street
Lymington, Hants

Edinburgh   D. Napier & Sons Ltd
                       17–18 Bristo Place
                       Edinburgh

Jersey   Norwegian Health Salon
                       6a La Motte Street
                       Jersey
                       Channel Islands

London   G. Baldwin
                       171–173 Walworth Road
                       London
                       SE17

                       Neal's Yard Apothecary
                       Neal's Yard
                       Covent Garden
                       London
                       WC2

Ryde   The Grail Pharmacy
                       The Collonade
                       Lind Street
                       Ryde
                       Isle of Wight

Sheffield   Wickers Health Stores
                       195 Cattle Market
                       Sheffield

Southampton   Cathay of Bournemouth Ltd
                       32–33 Hanover Buildings
                       Central Southampton

Culpeper Herbal Shops can be found in nine major towns,
including three in London.

Glossary of common medical terms

Very often when reading, or on having a medical consultation, words are used which may not be familiar. This short list will help to make some of the more common ones a little clearer.

Alterative	Any substance that can beneficially alter the condition of a patient.
Amenorrhoea	Cessation of the menstrual flow.
Anodyne	Any substance which eases pain.
Antiseptic	Any substance that prevents putrefaction.
Antispasmodic	Any substance that prevents or relieves spasms.
Anthelmintic	Any herb acting against intestinal worms.
Aperient	Any substance producing the natural evacuation of the bowels.
Aphrodisiac	Any substance that stimulates sexual functions.
Astringent	Any substance which causes contraction of body tissues.
Cardiac	Any condition affecting or pertaining to the heart.
Carminative	Any substance that relieves pain caused by flatulence.
Cathartic	Any substance that induces stimulation of bowel action; rather stronger than aperients.
Corrective	Any substance that restores normal conditions.

Debility	Feebleness of health.
Degenerative	Deterioration or change in tissue structure.
Demulcent	Any soothing medicine.
Deobstruent	Any substance that frees the natural orifices of the body.
Diaphoretic	Any substance inducing perspiration.
Diuretic	Any substance that increases the flow of urine.
Dysmenorrhoea	Excessive pain during menstruation.
Emetic	Any substance that causes vomitting.
Emmenagogue	Any drug that stimulates menstruation.
Emollient	Any substance that soothes and lubricates.
Expectorant	Any substance that helps to clear the chest of phlegm by coughing.
Haemostatic	Any substance that checks bleeding, aids the clotting of blood.
Hepatic	A substance which benefits the liver.
Insecticide	Any substance that is fatal to insects.
Laxative	Any substance that induces gentle, easy bowel action.
Leucorrhea	Any mucous discharge from female genitals.
Menorrhagia	Excessive flow in menstruation.
Myalgia	Any muscular rheumatic pain.
Narcotic	Any drug that induces stupor and insensibility.
Nephritis	Any drug that affects the kidneys.
Nervine	Any substance that restores the nerves to a normal tone.
Oxytocic	Any drug that contracts the uterus and hastens childbirth.
Pectoral	Any substance used to allay chest disorders.
Parturient	Any product used during childbirth.

Purgative   A strong laxative.

Resolvent   Any substance that reduces swelling.

Rubefacient   Any substance that produces inflammation of the skin.

Sedative   Any substance used to placate 'nerves'.

Soporific   Any substance used to promote sleep.

Stimulant   Any substance used to promote the reserve power of the body and produce strength and energy.

Stomachic   Any substance that allays stomach disorders.

Styptic   Any substance that aids the clotting of blood.

Sudorific   Any substance producing heavy perspiration.

Tonic   Any substance that, if used regularly, will promote vivacity and well being.

Vermifuge   Any substance that expels worms from the body.

Vulnerary   Any substance that promotes the healing of wounds.